SAFETY SMARTS

SAFE IN YOUR

HOME

PowerKiDS
press
New York

VICTOR BLAINE

Published in 2017 by The Rosen Publishing Group, Inc.
29 East 21st Street, New York, NY 10010

First Edition

Editor: Theresa Morlock
Book Design: Reann Nye

Photo Credits: Cover (background) Photographee.eu/Shutterstock.com; cover (boy) kurhan/Shutterstock.com; p. 5 Gary Burchell/Taxi/Getty Images; p. 6 pikselstock/Shutterstock.com; p. 9 goodluz/Shutterstock.com; p. 10 Blend Images/Shutterstock.com; pp. 13, 22 wavebreakmedia/Shutterstock.com; p. 14 Danaij/Shutterstock.com; p. 17 Teresa Short/Moment/Getty Images; p. 18 Fuse/Corbis/Getty Images; p. 21 Maskot/Getty Images; p. 24 (outlet) R. Roth/Shutterstock.com; p. 24 (stairs) ben bryant/Shutterstock.com; p. 24 (stove) Iriana Shiyan/Shutterstock.com.

Cataloging-in-Publication Data

Names: Blaine, Victor.
Title: Safe in your home / Victor Blaine.
Description: New York : PowerKids Press, 2017. | Series: Safety smarts | Includes index.
Identifiers: ISBN 9781499427875 (pbk.) | ISBN 9781499429909 (library bound) | ISBN 9781499428650 (6 pack)
Subjects: LCSH: Home accidents–Prevention–Juvenile literature.Children's accidents–Prevention–Juvenile literature.Safety education–Juvenile literature.
Classification: LCC HV675.5 B53 2017 | DDC 613.6–dc23

Manufactured in the United States of America

CPSIA Compliance Information: Batch #BW17PK: For Further Information contact Rosen Publishing, New York, New York at 1-800-237-9932

CONTENTS

Our home is special.

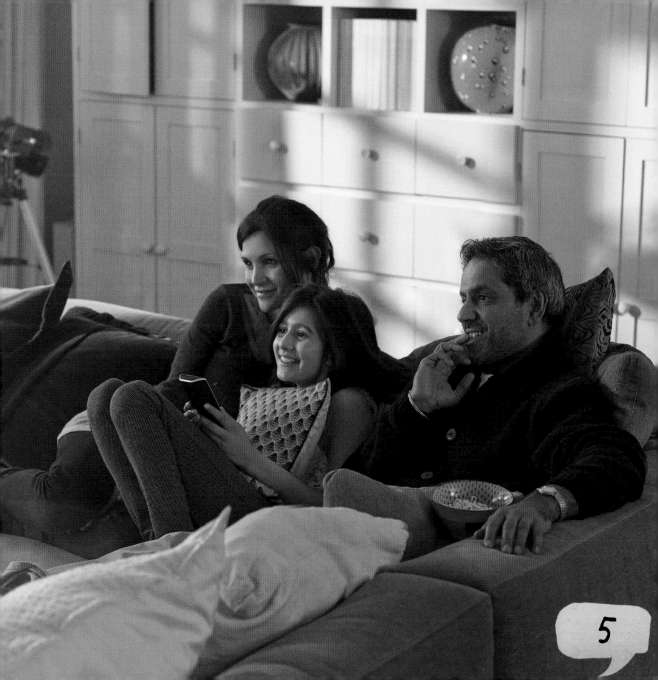

5

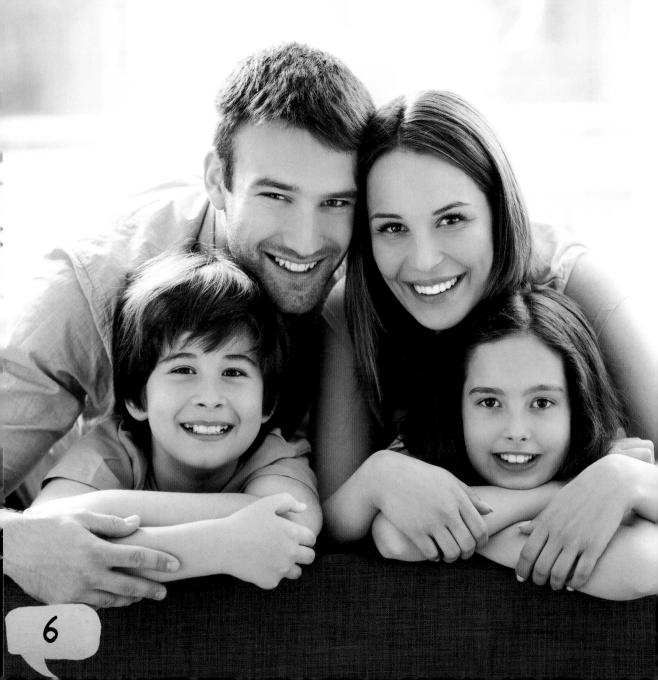

How can we stay safe?

Our parents answer the door.

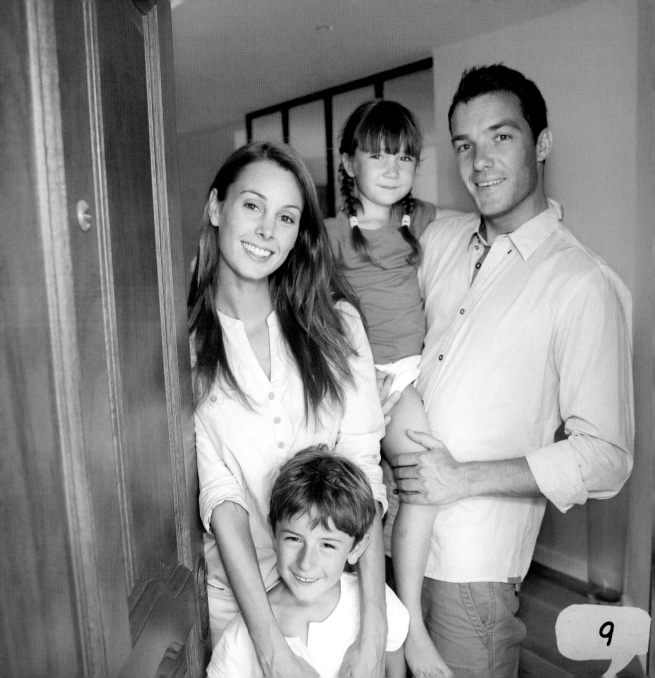

9

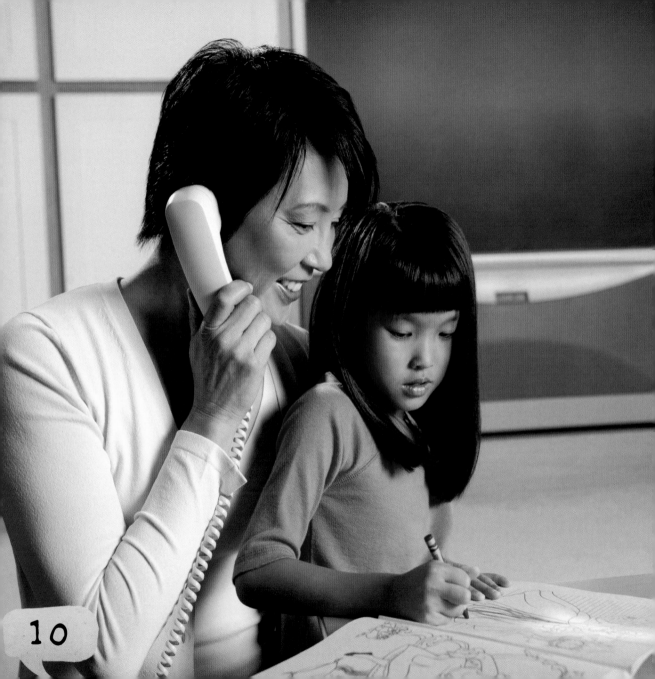

Our parents answer
the phone.

11

Sharp things can cut us.

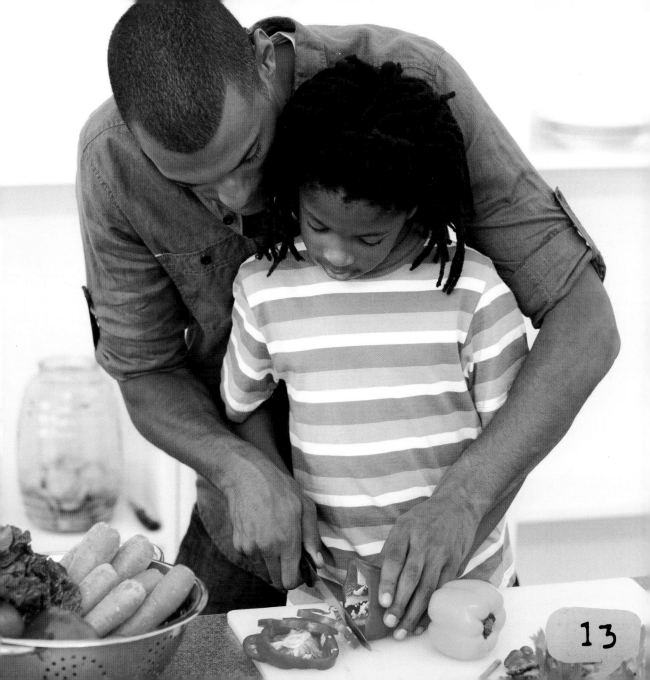

13

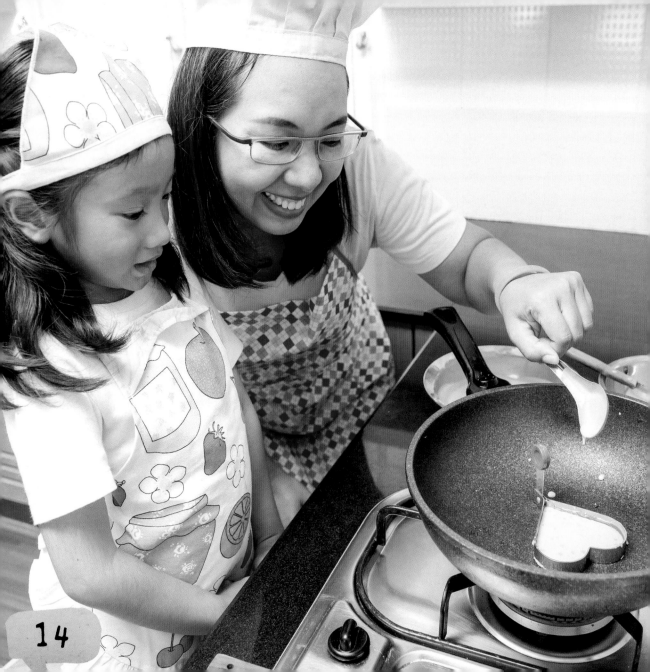

The **stove** can burn us.

Outlets can shock us!

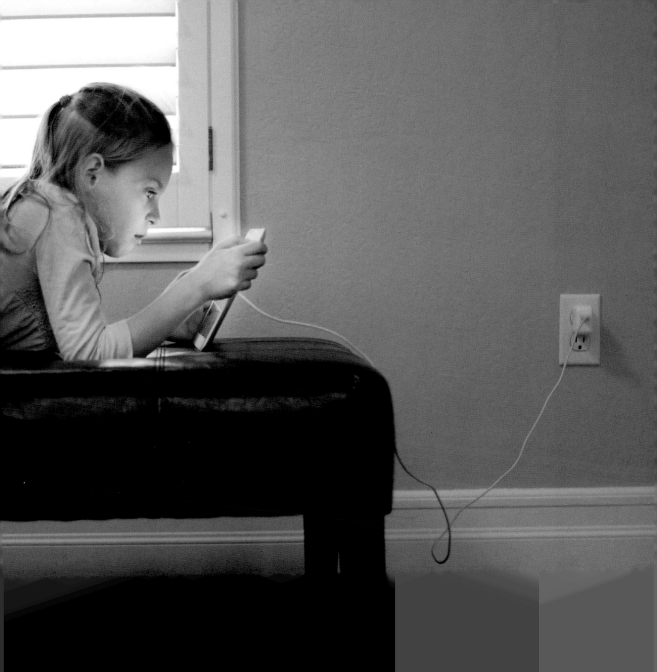

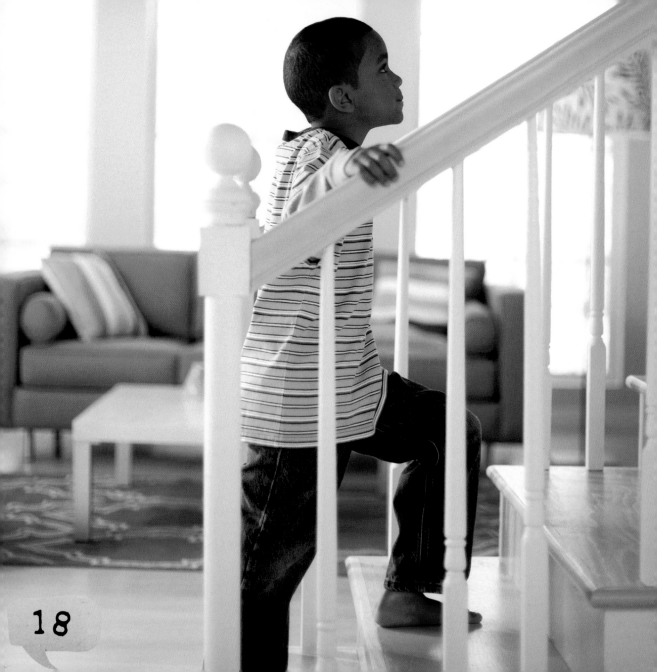

18

We walk on the **stairs**.

We clean up our toys.

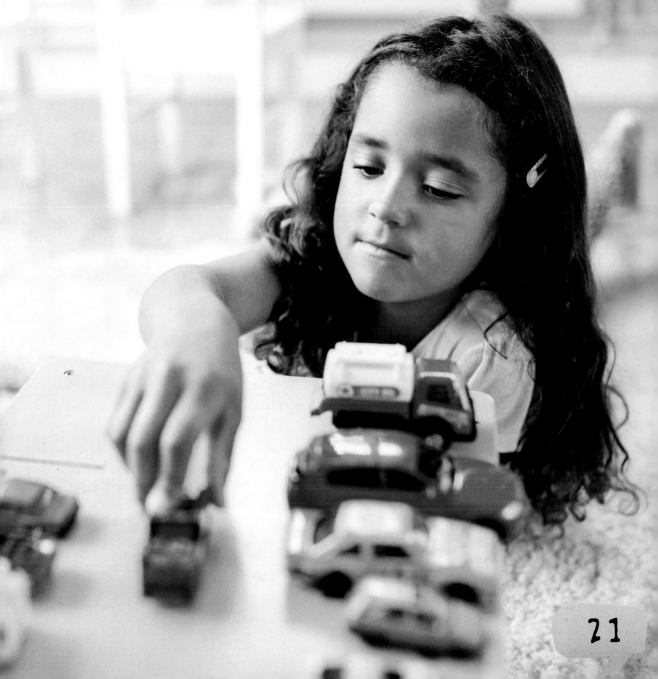

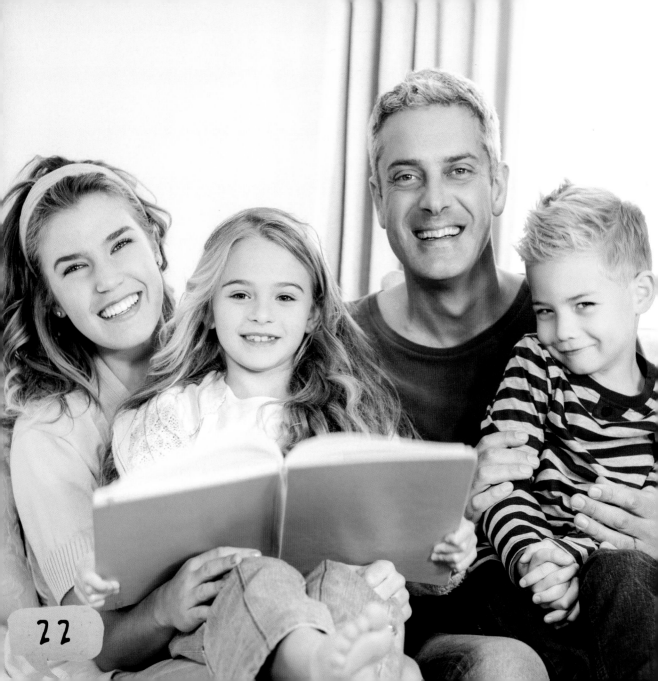

22

Our home is safe!

WORDS TO KNOW

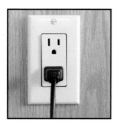

outlet

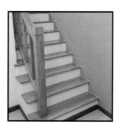

stairs

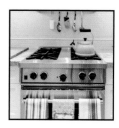

stove

INDEX

WEBSITES

Due to the changing nature of Internet links, PowerKids Press has developed an online list of websites related to the subject of this book. This site is updated regularly. Please use this link to access the list: www.powerkidslinks.com/safe/home